Hèla Ben Jmaà
Taieb Cherif
Mohamed Seddik

Surgery for triple valve disease

Hèla Ben Jmaà
Taieb Cherif
Mohamed Seddik

Surgery for triple valve disease

ScienciaScripts

Imprint

Any brand names and product names mentioned in this book are subject to trademark, brand or patent protection and are trademarks or registered trademarks of their respective holders. The use of brand names, product names, common names, trade names, product descriptions etc. even without a particular marking in this work is in no way to be construed to mean that such names may be regarded as unrestricted in respect of trademark and brand protection legislation and could thus be used by anyone.

Cover image: www.ingimage.com

This book is a translation from the original published under ISBN 978-620-6-71967-0.

Publisher:
Sciencia Scripts
is a trademark of
Dodo Books Indian Ocean Ltd. and OmniScriptum S.R.L publishing group

120 High Road, East Finchley, London, N2 9ED, United Kingdom
Str. Armeneasca 28/1, office 1, Chisinau MD-2012, Republic of Moldova, Europe
Printed at: see last page
ISBN: 978-620-7-98644-6

I- INTRODUCTION

Triple valve disease refers to dysfunction of the three heart valves: mitral, aortic and tricuspid. This condition is essentially of rheumatic origin [1].

These valvulopathies have now become rare in Western countries due to the decline in rheumatic fever (RF). However, they are still common in our country [2].

These triple disorders are characterised by a wide variety of clinical presentations and outcomes, as they combine varying degrees of leakage and stenosis in each of the valve orifices [3].

Diagnosis of this pathology relies essentially on cardiac Doppler ultrasound, which also allows an assessment of the impact on cardiac function and pulmonary pressures. The treatment of this condition has benefited greatly from advances in cardiac surgery over the last few decades. However, despite advances in surgical techniques, myocardial protection and post-operative resuscitation, this surgery is still associated with a high mortality rate [3, 4].

II- ANATOMICAL REMINDER

1- The mitral valve [5] :

The mitral valve system is a complex anatomical entity made up of several components that form a functional entity. These are the valve tissue, the mitral annulus, the tendinous cords and the papillary muscles or pillars. The cords and pillars make up the sub-valvular apparatus, which is involved in the systolic function of the LV. There are two valves: an anterior valve or large valve and a posterior valve or small valve; and two commissures: an anterolateral commissure and a posteromedial commissure.The anterior valve is semicircular in shape. Its attachment margin represents approximately two-fifths of the annular circumference. It is divided into three segments: A1: anterior commissural region, A2: medial region, A3: posterior commissural region. The posterior valve is quadrangular in shape. Its attachment margin represents three-fifths of the annular circumference. Its height is less than that of the anterior valve, so that the surface area of the two valves is identical. It is divided into three segments: P1: anterior commissural region, P2: medial region, P3: posterior commissural region.

Tendon cords are classified :

- Depending on the insertion height :

• Marginal or primary cords inserted on the free edges of the valves. They prevent valve prolapse.

• Intermediate or secondary cords inserted on the ventricular face of the valves.

• Basal cords inserted at the base of valve attachment

- Depending on the site of valve implantation :

• Commissural cords: there is one commissural cord per commissure

• Anterior valve cords: two cords inserted on the ventricular side of the valve

• Posterior valve cords

The papillary or pillar muscles: there are two pillars in the LV:
- The anterolateral pillar, consisting of a muscular head

- The posteromedial pillar is often composed of two muscular chiefs
The mitral annulus: this is the junction between the left atrium and the left ventricle. It inserts into the mitral valve tissue.

2- The aortic valve [6] :

The aortic valve is a much simpler structure than the atrioventricular valves: it closes under the effect of the diastolic pressure of the aorta without any subvalvular apparatus. The stress zones are the three valve commissures and the free edges of the three cusps, which constitute the coaptation zones. The aortic ring is scalloped: the attachment zone of the three cusps is high in relation to the commissures, with the valvular insertion descending very low towards the ventricle.Between the lower insertion zone of the middle part of the cusps and the upper insertion zone of the commissures, the sinuses of Valsalva develop opposite each of the cusps, designated according to the emergence of each of the two coronaries: right coronary sinus, left coronary sinus and non-coronary sinus. Several diameters therefore need to be taken into account in the dynamics of aortic flow: subaortic diameter (left ventricular outflow tract), diameter of the the annulus, diameter of the aorta at the level of the sinuses of Valsalva, diameter of the sino-tubular junction, and diameter of the ascending aorta downstream.

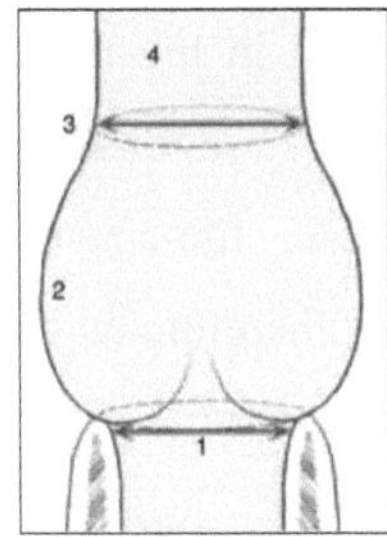

Figure 1: Diameters of the aortic ejection pathway [6].

1. Subaortic diameter (21 mm); 2. Sinus of Valsalva (33 mm);

3. Sinotubular junction (28 mm); 4. Ascending aorta (29.5 mm).

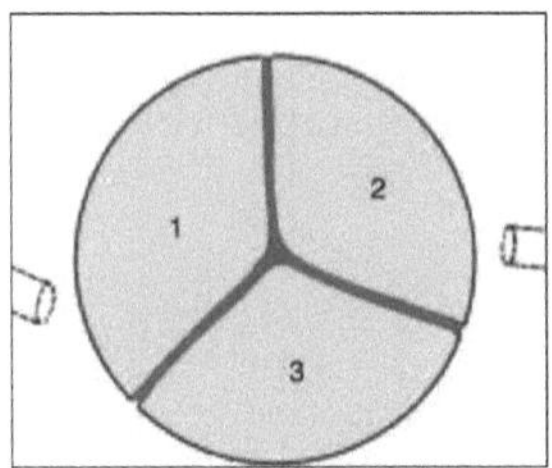

Figure 2: Superior view of the aortic valve [6].

1. Left coronary sinus; 2. right coronary sinus; 3. non-coronary sinus.

3- The tricuspid valve [7] :

The tricuspid valve consists of three leaflets: anterior, septal and posterior. The relationship between the tricuspid annulus and the atrioventricular conduction pathways is essential for reconstructive surgery or valve replacement. The atrioventricular node and the His bundle that follows it are located at the posterosuperior edge of the membranous septum. Koch's triangle is bounded by Todaro's tendon and the tricuspid annulus. Todaro's tendon is a linear structure stretched between the coronary sinus and the anteroseptal commissure.

The atrioventricular node is located in the corner of Koch's triangle between Todaro's tendon and the tricuspid annulus. Any traumatic lesion of the conduction tissue leads to complete, immediate and definitive atrioventricular block, requiring a pacemaker. It is therefore an area to be avoided, which is one of the particularities of tricuspid valve surgery.

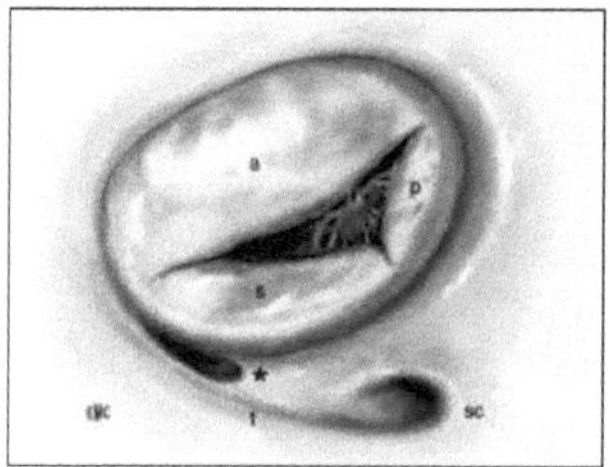

Figure 3: Anatomy of the tricuspid valve [7].

a: anterior leaflet; p: posterior leaflet; s: septal leaflet.

Location of conduction pathways: t: tendon of Todaro; *: sinus node. The tip of Koch's triangle lies between Todaro's tendon and the insertion of the septal leaflet. The sinus node is located in the apex and extends into the His bundle.

III-EPIDEMIOLOGY

1- Impact :

In view of the persistence of rheumatic heart disease, which is still common in our country [2], triple valvular disease remains a major health problem with a high risk of death. high morbidity and mortality. This pathological association has become rare in Western countries [1].

2- Age :

In the Mullany series [8], the average age is 54. In the Alsoufi series [3], it is 58.2 years, and 62 years in the Carrier series [4].

The mean age was 40 years in the series by Akay [9], 42 years in the series by Han [10], and 34.7 years in the series by Eukouhen [11].

In developing countries, this condition mainly affects young adults, unlike in developed countries where it occurs in an older population. The predominance of degenerative pathology in Western countries and rheumatic pathology in developing countries explains this significant age difference.

Table 1: Mean age of patients operated on for triple valve disease, by series.

series	Average age of patients (years)
Alsoufi [3]	58,2
Carrier [4]	62
Mullany (USA) [8]	54
Akay [9]	41,8
Han [10]	42
Eukouhen (Morocco-Casablanca) [11]	34,7

3- Gender :

The distribution of patients by sex shows a clear predominance of women in the series by Carrier [4] and Han [10], where the percentage of women is 63% and 75% respectively. This is explained by the predominance of rheumatic diseases in women.

IV- PATHOPHYSIOLOGY [12, 13]

Each type of valve damage has an effect on the heart chambers, the systemic circulation, the pulmonary circulation and other valve structures. These effects can interact in different ways. For example, the effects of one type of valve damage may minimise the consequences of another or, on the contrary, aggravate them.

1- Mitral stenosis :

Mitral stenosis is an obstacle to left atrioventricular blood flow during diastole.

*1.1.*Consequences downstream :

Left ventricular pressure was normal.

*1.2.*Consequences upstream :

The mean pressure in the left atrium is increased, giving rise to a mean trans-mitral diastolic gradient, the value of which depends on the degree of stenosis [14]. The increase in left atrial pressure will progressively affect all the structures located upstream of the mitral valve: The left atrium gradually dilates. Its wall gradually alters and thins, and fibrous tissue replaces the muscle fibres. The increase in pressure is transmitted to the veins, the pulmonary capillaries and then the pulmonary arteries, resulting in post-capillary PAH, which is reversible with treatment, and irreversible pre-capillary PAH. The impact on the right heart first manifests itself as right ventricular hypertrophy, followed by dilatation and heart failure with functional tricuspid insufficiency.

2- Mitral insufficiency :

Mitral insufficiency is an abnormal reflux of blood from the left ventricle into the left atrium during systole. The consequences depend on the volume of regurgitation and whether the leak is acute or chronic.

2.1. Consequences downstream :

Volume overload initially leads to an increase in the workload of the left ventricle. Over time, this leads to dilatation and left ventricular failure, resulting in a drop in systemic flow.

2.2. Consequences upstream :

When regurgitation becomes chronic, the left atrium dilates and becomes more complicated. Left atrial pressure is normal or slightly elevated. The pulmonary circulation and right ventricle are then affected, with functional tricuspid insufficiency.

3- Aortic stenosis :

Aortic stenosis creates a systolic obstacle to ejection from the left ventricle to the aorta.

3.1. Consequences downstream :

Circulatory conditions (cardiac output, aortic pressure) remain unchanged until an advanced stage, involving a lengthening of left ventricular ejection time, an increase in ejection velocity, and a systolic pressure gradient that is greater the tighter the stenosis. In the case of narrow aortic stenosis, cardiac output remains normal at rest for a long time, then increases insufficiently on exertion, which explains the symptoms on exertion (syncope, angina, dyspnoea).

3.2. **Consequences upstream :**

Upstream, there is concentric hypertrophy of the left ventricle, then at a later stage, left ventricular failure occurs, leading to dilatation of the LV and a reduction in cardiac output. The final stage is right ventricular failure and functional tricuspid insufficiency.

3.3. **Coronary circulation :**

Insufficient coronary flow during exercise and increased oxygen requirements due to left ventricular hypertrophy are factors that can lead to exertional angina.

4- Aortic insufficiency :

Aortic insufficiency is a diastolic reflux of blood from the aorta into the left ventricle. In chronic aortic insufficiency, the LV is subjected to a simultaneous increase in preload and afterload. It adapts to these new load conditions through progressive remodelling involving dilatation and hypertrophy [15]. At this stage of compensation, the LV is a dilated, hypertrophied, compliant cavity, capable of providing a large ejection volume without upstream repercussions on the pulmonary circulation.At a later stage of decompensation, the LV continues to dilate and its mass to increase. Its compliance decreases and its ejection fraction falls [15].

5- Tricuspid narrowing [12] :

Tricuspid stenosis obstructs the flow of blood from the right atrium to the right ventricle during diastole, resulting in a diastolic pressure gradient between the right atrium and the right ventricle. It does not exceed the gradient of mitral stenosis, which usually coexists with tricuspid stenosis. Mitral stenosis leads to a fall in right heart rate, which tends to reduce the tricuspid gradient. This decrease is marked in the case of tight double stenosis, and may mask the haemodynamic signs of the tricuspid obstruction. The increase in right atrial pressure is transmitted upstream, explaining the turgidity of the jugular veins. Tricuspid narrowing also plays a relatively protective role against paroxysmal pulmonary events in mitral stenosis.

6- Tricuspid insufficiency [13] :

Tricuspid insufficiency is characterised by systolic right ventriculoatrial regurgitation. Functional tricuspid insufficiency secondary to dilatation of the annulus is contrasted with organic insufficiency due to damage to the leaflets, cords or pillars. Tricuspid insufficiency increases right ventricular preload. It thus contributes to ventricular dilatation. Right atrial pressure rises as a result of increased ventricular filling pressure and, above all, systolic regurgitation. The right atrium dilates and the atrial hyperpressure is transmitted upstream to the systemic venous circulation.

7- Polyvalvulopathies [13] :

Upstream stenosis protects the heart chamber or chambers between the two attacks from the impact of downstream valvulopathy. When severe mitral stenosis is combined with severe aortic insufficiency, mitral stenosis will reduce ventricular filling, reducing the impact of aortic insufficiency on left ventricular volume, which will be slightly dilated [16]. Conversely, downstream stenosis will worsen the consequences of upstream organic regurgitation. For example, severe aortic stenosis will worsen the degree of mitral insufficiency [17]. The presence of two successive stenoses downstream and upstream of the left ventricle protects the latter from the impact of aortic stenosis, or at least reduces its clinical expression and haemodynamic consequences [18]. On the contrary, the combination of aortic insufficiency and mitral insufficiency will impose a volumetric overload on the left ventricle due to both aortic regurgitation and increased left atrioventricular flow, resulting in significant dilatation of the left ventricle [18].

V- ETIOLOGIES

1- Rheumatic fever :

Triple valve damage is mostly rheumatic in origin. Most often, they correspond to a combination of mitro-aortic valve disease and functional tricuspid insufficiency, and more rarely to triple organic damage [19].

1.1. **Pathogenesis [20] :**

Rheumatic disease is caused by group A beta-haemolytic streptococcus. It appears as a delayed, non-suppurative complication of streptococcal infection. It is currently considered to be the result of an immune conflict in the cellular state.

1.2. **Frequency [19] :**

The prevalence of rheumatic carditis in developing countries is high.

Paradoxically, in developed countries, AARS has become rare since the 1970s. A resurgence of a few sporadic outbreaks has been noted since 1987, in connection with the phenomenon of migration.

1.3. **Pathological anatomy [19] :**

- Mitral valve lesions :

Involvement of the mitral valve involves the valvular and subvalvular apparatus:

- Lesions of the valve leaflets: the valves are altered to varying degrees: thickened then sclerotic, sometimes calcified. The mobility and suppleness of the valves, especially the posterior valve, disappears, resulting in advanced forms of the form of a rigid funnel. Calcifications are inconstant. They may involve the free edge or the body of the valves.

- Lesions of the commissures: The characteristic lesion is more or less complete symphysis of the commissures. The valves are thus fused and the mitral orifice is often oval-shaped and has a reduced surface area.

- Damage to the subvalvular apparatus: the cords are thickened, fused and shortened. These changes can lead to isolated mitral narrowing, mitral disease or, more rarely, isolated mitral insufficiency.

- Aortic valve lesions :

Lesions are characterised by the fusion of one, two or three commissures over a variable area, and by the thickening and retraction of the sigmoid. The aortic orifice is therefore rounded or triangular in shape, forming a more or less severe stenosis which is usually associated with regurgitation. Calcifications affect the commissures and sigmoid.The restricted movement of the aortic sigmoid resulting from these changes leads to aortic narrowing, insufficiency or disease.

- Lesions of the tricuspid valve :

Tricuspid involvement may be organic, of rheumatic origin, or functional, in the event of repercussions on right ventricular function:

- Organic tricuspid disorder: the lesions responsible are commissural fusion with thickening and retraction of the valve leaflets and sub-valvular apparatus, resulting in a more or less significant reduction in valve mobility. This organic damage most often leads to tricuspid disease, more rarely to stenosis or isolated tricuspid insufficiency.

- Functional tricuspid disorder: by dilation and deformation of the annulus without any real macroscopic organic damage.

1. 4 Prevention :

Preventing RAA is the only way to reduce the morbidity and mortality of rheumatic valve disease. Prevention is based on :

- Early treatment of angina

- Integrating the fight against AAR into the primary healthcare programme at individual and community level

RAA prophylaxis can be carried out at various levels:

- Primary prevention even before the onset of AAR

- Secondary prevention of RAA to avoid relapses and progression to rheumatic heart disease.

2- Dystrophic and degenerative diseases :

Dystrophic disease is a source of distension. They may be secondary to dystrophy of the valvular elastic fibres responsible for a double mitro-aortic leak, particularly in Marfan's disease [21].

Degenerative lesions lead to progressive calcification of the valve apparatus, which in elderly patients is responsible for calcified aortic narrowing (sometimes associated with coronary damage) and organic mitral leakage. These lesions are associated with functional tricuspid insufficiency.

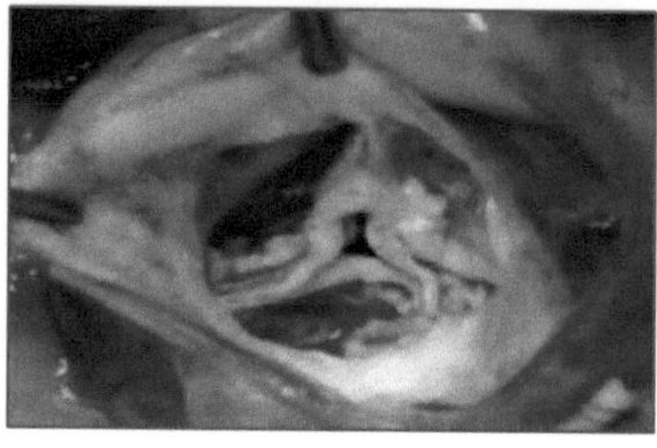

Figure 4: Macroscopic appearance of a degenerative calcified aortic valve [6].

3- Infective endocarditis [19] :

Triple endocardial disease is exceptional. Valvular lesions take the form of vegetations of varying size. In the aortic sigmoid, they are located on the ventricular side, whereas in the mitral leaflets, they are located on the atrial side. Trans-oesophageal ultrasound is required to recognise them. These vegetations are associated with destructive lesions such as perforation and tearing of the aortic or mitral valves, as well as para-valvular lesions such as abscesses. In the series by Alsoufi [3], the aetiology of valvulopathy was AR in 10% of cases.

The clinical expression of polyvalvulopathies is highly polymorphic and depends on many factors. The main factors are the location of each lesion, its type (leak, stenosis, or a combination of the two), its degree and whether it is organic or functional [19]. The coexistence of the three conditions can lead to the clinical expression of one of them being minimised or the natural course of the disease being altered.

1- Dyspnoea [19] :

The predominant functional symptomatology in most patients is dyspnoea at an advanced stage.

Table XIII shows the results of some published series.

Table 2: Functional stage of patients according to studies.

series	Year	Stage II	Stage III	Stage IV
Yilmaz [20]	2004	23,5%	64,7%	11,8%
Alsoufi [3]	2006	6%	48%	46%
Han [10]	2007	15%	56%	29%
Berriane [21]	2009	7,8%	70,5%	21,7%

In the majority of cases, valvulopathy is at an advanced stage of the disease, which can be explained by a delay in treatment. This delay is often linked to the refusal of surgery or a lack of resources.

2- Angina :

Acar [22] reported 27.3% cases of angina in his series.

3- Palpitations :

This symptomatology was not marked in several series. These palpitations are most often associated with supraventricular rhythm disorders frequently observed in cases of mitral stenosis. This was the case in our series where mitral pathology was predominant due to ARF.

4. Signs of right heart failure :

In addition to dyspnoea, the signs of right heart failure reflect the progression of the disease. This was observed in most of the series reviewed, in particular that of Berriane [21], where 49% of patients had signs of heart failure. In Han's series [10], the rate of right heart failure was 38%.

VII- ADDITIONAL TESTS

1- Chest X-ray :

Radiologically, cardiomegaly was identified in all patients in Goutandji's series [23].

2- Electrocardiogram :

Atrial fibrillation is a major complication of valve disease. This is explained by the impact of valve damage on the left atrium, which is usually dilated or even ectatic.This is explained by the importance of mitral pathology (rheumatic origin), compared with Western countries where aortic valve disease (degenerative origin) is predominant.Table III shows the frequency of CA/FA in some published series.

Table III: Frequency of CA/FA by series.

series	Year	Frequency of CA/FA
Berriane [21]	2009	69%
Han [10]	2007	47%
Akay [9]	2006	40,8%
Yilmaz [20]	2004	26%

3- Trans-thoracic echocardiography :

As part of the assessment of lesions in the disease, TTE is the reference examination. It is used to confirm the diagnosis, determine the severity of valve damage and its impact on left ventricular function and pulmonary circulation.

3.1. **Positive diagnosis :**

The results vary according to the series: Han [10] found a majority of mitral narrowing and Garg [24] found a majority of mitral insufficiency. In Alsoufi's series [3], patients were evenly divided between mitral narrowing, insufficiency and disease. Concerning the aortic valve, the frequency of aortic disease was 48.5%, and that of isolated aortic leakage was 34.2%, in the series by Garg [24] and Alsoufi [3].

As regards tricuspid valve pathology, a predominance of tricuspid insufficiency has been observed in all the series studied [3, 24].

At an advanced stage of the disease, triple valvulopathy is likely to have an impact on the heart chambers, particularly the LV, on the ejection fraction and on the pulmonary circulation, reflecting the poor prognosis of the disease:

3.2. **Impact on cardiac function :**

❖ **LV end-diastolic diameter :**

In the series by Yilamz [20], the LV was dilated in 54.2% of cases, with a mean DTD of 56.2 mm.

❖ **LV ejection fraction :**

Through complex pathophysiological mechanisms, the LV dilates and its ejection fraction progressively decreases. This was found in Han's series, where 66% of patients had reduced systolic function with an LVEF < 50% [10].

3.3. **Impact on the pulmonary circulation :**

Left-sided valve damage has an impact on the pulmonary circulation.

4- Coronary angiography :

The indications for this examination were the same in all the articles, two of which are major:

✓ Age > 40.

✓ LV dysfunction.

VIII- TREATMENT

1- Pre-operative assessment :

In Han's series [10], 16% of patients were hypertensive and 11% had diabetes.

2- Approach :

The classic approach currently used by most surgeons is the median sternotomy. It allows rapid and easy installation of the CEC, and access to all the cardiac cavities. This approach was demonstrated in all series.

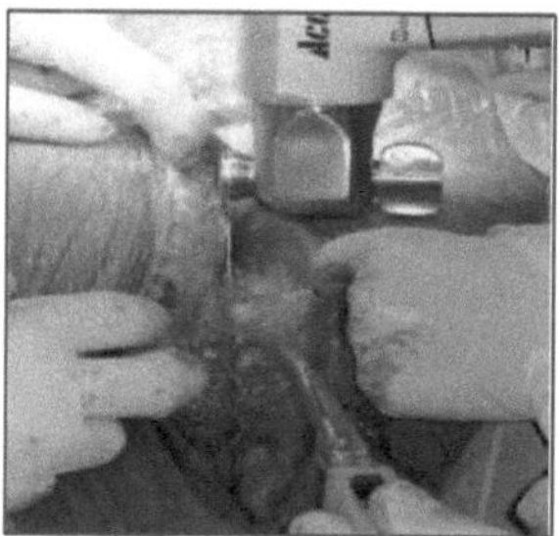

Figure 5: Vertical median sternotomy [25].

3- Extracorporeal circulation :

Normothermia was the rule in our daily practice. In fact, several authors have advocated the advantages of this technique over hypothermia, with less inflammatory reaction and better control of haemostasis. This results in fewer post-operative complications [26]. However, according to Vazquez-Jimenez et al [27], moderate hypothermia during cardiac surgery can significantly reduce myocardial cell damage and myocardial cell death.

Table IV: Mean duration of bypass surgery and aortic clamping according to series.

series	Year	Duration of CEC (min)	Aortic clamping time (min)
Berriane [21]	2009	174	136
Han [10]	2007	147	115
Alsoufi [3]	2006	158	123
Carrier [4]	2002	184	143

4- Valve approaches :

4.1. Aortic valve [6] :

The aortotomy is performed as a "hockey stick", with a transverse opening on the anterior surface approximately 15 mm downstream of the origin of the right coronary artery. On the left, the incision continues upwards towards the pulmonary artery, and on the right, the incision descends obliquely towards the middle of the non-coronary sinus, stopping 10 mm from the annulus.

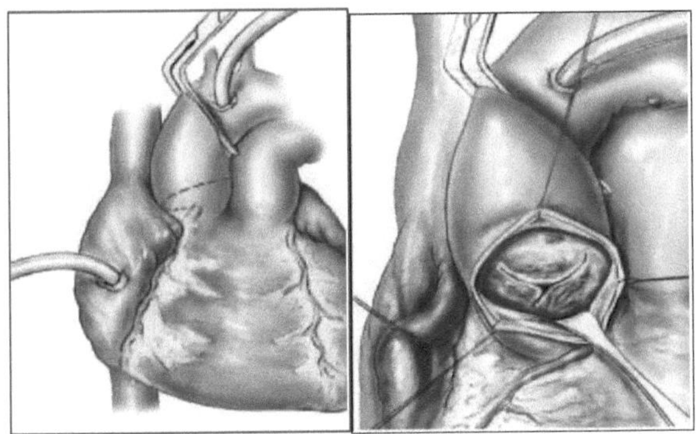

Figure 6: Hockey stick aortotomy [6].

4.2. Mitral valve [5] :

The left auriculotomy is the approach to the mitral valve parallel to the atrial groove or Sondergaardt's groove. The surgical approach is a long incision parallel to the atrial groove and 2 cm behind it.

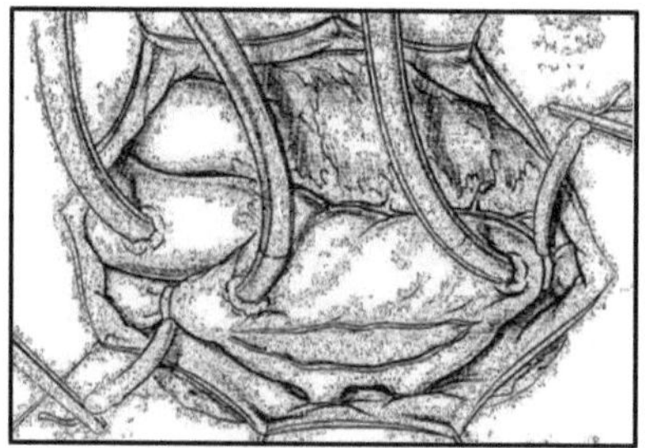

Figure 7: Approach to the left atrium via an incision parallel to Sondergaardt's sulcus [5].

4.3. Tricuspid valve :

The incision in the atrium is made in front of the cannulae, parallel to the atrioventricular groove, which facilitates analysis because the tricuspid valve is superficial.

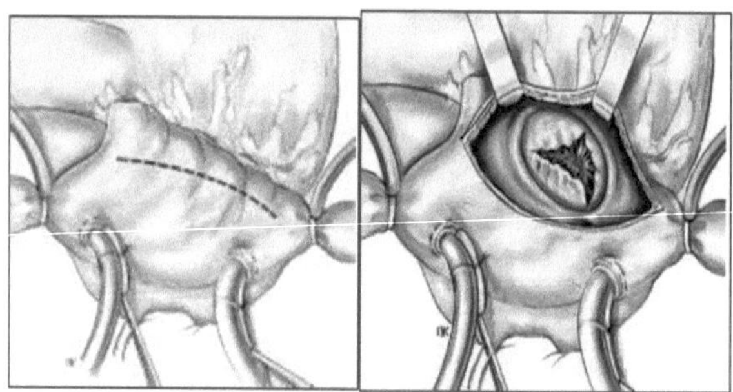

Figure 8: Right auriculotomy [7].

5- Valve procedures :

5.1. Aortic valve :

During aortic valve replacement, exposure of the valve is provided by placing a retractor over the lower lip of the aortotomy. The first stage of the operation is an analysis of the valvular lesion of the aortic arch and the orifices. coronary arteries. The second stage involves resection of the valve. This is an important and delicate procedure that must be carried out with great care and attention to avoid disseminating friable calcareous debris into the aorta, left ventricle and coronary arteries [6]. The third step is choosing the prosthesis. In order to assess the choice of diameter, the three commissural stitches are inserted using splayed "U" stitches. The final stage involves fitting the prosthesis and securing it with simple or U-shaped stitches. Before closing the aortotomy, it is always necessary to check that there is no periprosthetic dehiscence, that the prosthesis is correctly inserted on the ring and that the coronary orifices are free. Aortic valve replacement was the rule in all series except that of Alsoufi [3], where 8% of patients underwent aortic valve plasty. The indications for plastic surgery have not yet been proven to be effective in the long term, particularly in the case of rheumatic diseases and acquired aortic valve disease in adults [19].

5.2. Mitral valve :

- Mitral valve replacement: After the retractor has been placed for exposure, the anterior valve is secured in the middle near its free edge by a traction wire, which allows the scissors or scalpel to be used around the entire circumference until the valve tissue has been completely removed. The posterior valve is almost always preserved.

This significantly reduces the risk of rupture of the free wall of the left ventricle. The size of the valve is selected using a special measuring device. The orientation of the valve is then important. The anti-anatomical position provides the best haemodynamic performance post-operatively.

Finally, the valve is attached using separate single or U-shaped stitches.

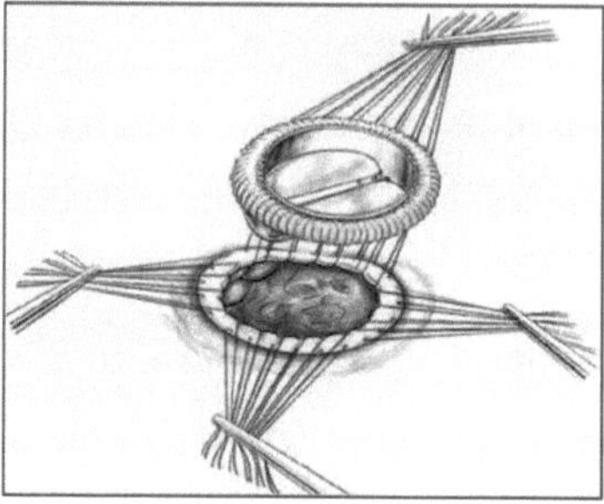

Figure 9: Schematic view of mitral valve replacement by mechanical prosthesis [5].

- Conservative surgery of the mitral valve: Despite advances in surgery and improvements in surgical techniques allowing greater conservation of the mitral sub-valvular apparatus, mitral valvuloplasty remains the only technique that truly respects the sub-valvular apparatus, but it is not always feasible [28].
The indications for mitral plasty are limited in the case of rheumatic valvulopathy due to changes and calcifications of the leaflets and cords [29].
In the case of infective endocarditis, the extent of valve abscesses determines the possibility of repair [30].

5.3. Tricuspid valve :

Another important issue to consider when evaluating a patient with triple valve disease is the tricuspid approach:

❖ Should it be replaced or kept?

❖ What type of annuloplasty would give the best long-term results?

❖ Between bioprosthesis and mechanical prosthesis, which would give the best results?

- **Annuloplasty using a prosthetic ring:** The aim is to restore the tricuspid annulus to its normal size and shape. The ring stitches are placed around the entire periphery of the ring except in the area of the His bundle. At the end of the procedure, a water test is carried out by injecting physiological saline into the right ventricle to check for leaks.

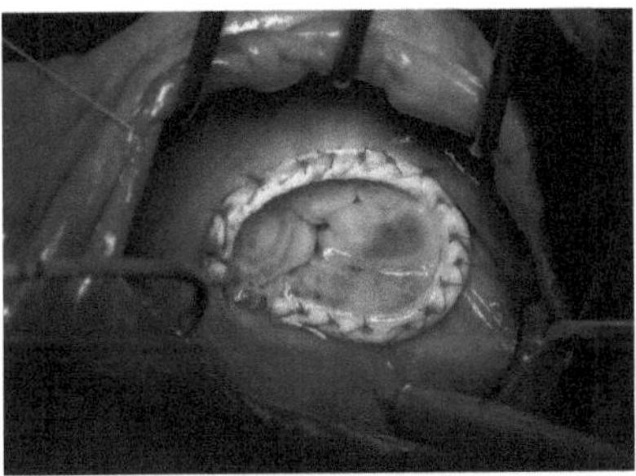

Figure 10: Annuloplasty using a prosthetic ring [31].

- **De Vega annuloplasty: This** is a reduction in the diameter of the tricuspid annulus using an over and under suture. A felt splint is placed at each end of the suture to try to prevent progressive tearing of the ring.

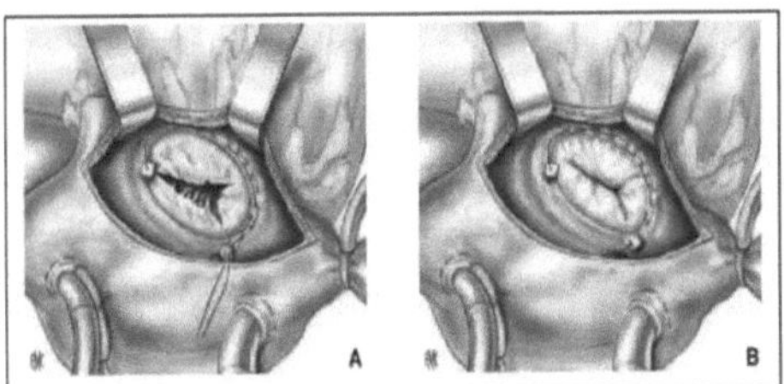

Figure 11: De Vega technique [32].

A: An overjet supported on felt is passed through the ring except in the septal area.

B: When the overlock is tightened, the diameter of the ring depends on the degree of tightening.

In the literature, tricuspidoplasty is preferred. However, the type of tricuspid valve replacement is not yet codified. Several authors believe that prosthetic tricuspid rings have a definite advantage in providing optimal stability to the repair [4]. De Vega annuloplasty is still favoured by some teams [1, 4, 33, 34]. Its advantages are the absence of foreign material, and therefore a very low economic cost, and a shorter aortic clamping time than prosthetic annuloplasty [35, 36]. However, it requires at least a reduction in the diameter of the tricuspid annulus, which must be less than 30 mm to obtain perfect continence [37]. In addition, the risk of progressive tearing of the annulus and disappearance of the suture remains high despite the suture being reinforced with felt [38].

- **Tricuspid valve replacement :** Excision of the tricuspid valve must respect the area of the anteroseptal commissure and the anterior part of the septal valve. In this way, trauma to the His bundle is avoided and tissue is preserved for suturing the valve substitute, whatever its type.

Some teams have chosen to carry out tricuspid valve replacement in cases of tricuspid disease, in cases of tricuspid insufficiency without PAH and in cases of re-operation on the tricuspid valve [20]. Experience of valve replacement in the tricuspid position remains limited and the choice between bioprosthesis and mechanical prosthesis remains controversial [9]. Some authors have found excellent results with bioprostheses in relation to their anti-thorombogenic characteristics with a better durability [39, 40]. Nevertheless, with the new generations of double-finned mechanical prostheses, several teams have demonstrated satisfactory results in the tricuspid position [41, 42]. In this context, Akay et al [9] hypothesised that when double mitro-aortic valve replacement with mechanical prostheses is planned, a third mechanical prosthesis in the tricuspid position would be a better choice. On the one hand, these patients require anticoagulation regardless of the type of prosthesis in the tricuspid position. On the other hand, in patients who have already undergone surgery, any potential re-intervention, in relation to bioprosthesis degeneration, should be avoided because of the increased operative risk. In summary, tricuspid plasty was the technique of choice in most series [9, 10, 20, 43].**[44]:**

6- Surgical indications :

*6.1.***Recommendations of the European Society of Cardiology 2012**

According to the Guidelines of the European Society of Cardiology published at According to the European Heart Journal 2012, [44] the indications for triple valve surgery are :

❖ When narrowing or insufficiency predominates, the indication follows the recommendations for the predominant valve damage.

❖ If the severity of the valve insufficiency or narrowing is the same, the indication for intervention should be based on the symptoms and objective consequences.

❖ In addition to the separate evolution of each valve lesion, it is necessary to take into account the interaction between the different lesions. This highlights the need to combine the various measurements, including assessment of the valve using methods that are less dependent on load conditions, such as planimetry.

❖ The indications for intervention are based on an overall assessment of the consequences of the various valve lesions, in particular the clinical symptoms and the impact on LV function.

❖ The decision to operate on several valves should take into account the additional surgical risk of combined procedures.

*6.2.***American Heart Association /American College of Cardiology recommendations 2014 [45]:**

According to the recommendations of the American College of Cardiology/American Heart Association published in the Journal of the

American College of Cardiology [45], the indications for triple valve surgery are:

❖ In the context of polyvalvular disease and in cases of mixed valve damage (insufficiency and narrowing), the indication for surgery should follow the recommendations for the predominant valve lesion. This consideration must be made with attention to :

• Clinical symptoms

• The severity of injuries

• Ventricular remodelling

• Surgical risk

• Result of the planned intervention

❖ The timing of the operation must take into account the coexistence of mixed disease (insufficiency + narrowing) and polyvalvular disease, which may have additional pathological consequences.

❖ For patients with moderate (non-severe) polyvalvulopathy, the timing of the operation is different. The operation may be indicated when there is :

• Clinical signs

• Pathophysiological consequences (reduced cardiac output, increased atrial and ventricular pressures).

6.3. **Indications for tricuspid surgery [42] :**

Tricuspid surgery must be performed early to avoid irreversible right ventricular dysfunction. Whenever technically possible, tricuspid plasty is preferred to valve replacement. According to ESC recommendations [44], the indications for surgery are :

❖ Severe symptomatic tricuspid narrowing.

❖ Severe tricuspid narrowing, if left heart surgery is envisaged.

❖ Moderate primary or secondary tricuspid insufficiency, if left heart surgery is envisaged.

❖ Insufficiency tricuspid insufficiency primary isolated severe without right ventricular dysfunction.

❖ Mild or moderate secondary tricuspid insufficiency with annulus dilatation ≥ 40 mm, if left heart surgery is being considered.

❖ Isolated asymptomatic or mildly symptomatic severe primary tricuspid insufficiency with impaired right ventricular function.

❖ Persistent or recurrent severe tricuspid insufficiency after left heart surgery in symptomatic patients or those with right ventricular dysfunction.

Table 16   Indications for tricuspid valve surgery

	Class[a]	Level[b]
Surgery is indicated in symptomatic patients with severe TS.[c]	I	C
Surgery is indicated in patients with severe TS undergoing left-sided valve intervention.[d]	I	C
Surgery is indicated in patients with severe primary or secondary TR undergoing left-sided valve surgery.	I	C
Surgery is indicated in symptomatic patients with severe isolated primary TR without severe right ventricular dysfunction.	I	C
Surgery should be considered in patients with moderate primary TR undergoing left-sided valve surgery.	IIa	C
Surgery should be considered in patients with mild or moderate secondary TR with dilated annulus (≥40 mm or >21 mm/m²) undergoing left-sided valve surgery.	IIa	C
Surgery should be considered in asymptomatic or mildly symptomatic patients with severe isolated primary TR and progressive right ventricular dilatation or deterioration of right ventricular function.	IIa	C
After left-sided valve surgery, surgery should be considered in patients with severe TR who are symptomatic or have progressive right ventricular dilatation/dysfunction, *in the absence* of left-sided valve dysfunction, severe right or left ventricular dysfunction, and severe pulmonary vascular disease.	IIa	C

PMC = percutaneous mitral commissurotomy; TR = tricuspid regurgitation;
TS = tricuspid stenosis
[a]Class of recommendation.
[b]Level of evidence.
[c]Percutaneous balloon valvuloplasty can be attempted as a first approach if TS is isolated.
[d]Percutaneous balloon valvuloplasty can be attempted if PMC can be performed on the mitral valve.

Figure 12: Indications for tricuspid surgery (ESC 2012 recommendations) [44].

1- Early results :

In general, the literature describes a high mortality rate of between 20% and 25% for tri-valvular surgery [46, 47]. However, some series have reported better results, with in-hospital mortality ranging from 8% to 17% [4, 10]. In order to reduce the incidence of postoperative low cardiac output, a new patient preparation protocol has been established using LEVOSIMENDAN in cases of LVEF < 40%. This drug is administered intravenously 24 hours before the operation and maintained for 24 to 48 hours afterwards. In addition, the Anaesthesia-Resuscitation team must maintain a protocol for early extubation of patients, adequate post-operative monitoring and early first lifting between D3 and D4 post-operatively. This will shorten the length of stay in intensive care, notably by reducing the rate of respiratory and infectious complications.

Table V: Operative mortality by series.

series	Number of patients	Year	Hospital mortality
Bourezak [48]	90	1984	37%
Donald [49]	90	1989	28,6%
Bortolotti [50]	453	1991	19%
Brown [51]	63	1993	31%
John [52]	456	2000	9,2%
Alsoufi [3]	174	2002	12,6%
Carrier [4]	73	2002	17%
Akay [9]	157	2006	2,5%
Han [10]	871	2007	8%
Yilmaz [20]	34	2007	11,8%
Pagni [53]	131	2013	10,6%

Certain risk factors for in-hospital mortality have been identified, such as the indication for urgent surgery in the series by Stephenson et al [54]. Some authors, such as Alsoufi [3] and Fadel [55], were unable to identify independent risk factors.

Table VI: Independent risk factors according to different series in the literature.

Risk factors	Han [10]	Carrier [4]	Akay [9]	Alsoufi [3]	Pagni [53]
NYHA IV	+	-	+	-	+
LV EF <50	+	-	+	-	-
DTD>50mm	-	-	+	-	-
Age> 50	-	+	-	-	-
IRC	-	-	-	-	+
EuroSCORE >5	-	-	-	-	-
Severe PAH	-	-	-	-	-

Early postoperative complications were comparable in most series. Infectious pneumopathy was marked in the series by Alsoufi [3] (15%), and the series by Akay [9] (3.1%). This could be due to an early extubation protocol and systematic preventive antibiotic therapy.

Table VII: Independent risk factors according to different series in the literature.

Complications	Alsoufi [3]	Akay [9]
Resumption for bleeding	6%	4,4%
Infectious lung disease	15%	3,1%
Sepsis	6%	3,4%
Renal insufficiency	4%	7%
Tamponade	4%	1,2%
Low cardiac output	6%	7%
Wall infection	2%	2,5%

2- Long-term monitoring :

- **Clinical follow-up:** Dyspnoea is the main symptom of the disease.

In the series by Carrier [4], 88% of patients were at NYHA stage I or II. However, these results were not found in the series by Alsoufi [3] (29% of patients retained stage II dyspnoea, 25% stage III, and 2% NYHA stage IV).

- **Ultrasound monitoring:** TTE is the reference para-clinical examination during post-operative monitoring of triple valve surgery. On the one hand, this examination makes it possible to detect any post-operative complications that may arise, and on the other, it enables the evolution of the disease to be monitored. However, the De Vega technique is often preferred by certain teams [3, 9, 10, 43] due to the speed with which it can be performed. This saves time, particularly during aortic clamping. Other teams [44] prefer prosthetic annuloplasty because of its greater durability.

- **Long-term survival:** Actuarial survival rates have been found in more recent literature.

Improved peri-operative management, including extensive experience of valve surgery, improved myocardial protection and post-operative care, have contributed to the excellent long-term survival results in this type of surgery.

Stage IV of the NYHA classification has been identified by several authors [9, 45, 46] as a factor significantly influencing long-term survival, as has severe PAH reported by Pagni et al [53] and chronic renal failure reported by Stephenson et al [54].

Table VIII: Survival at 5 and 10 years according to recent series.

Series	Number of patients	Years	Survival to 5 years	Survival to 10 years
Carrier [4]	73	2002	75%	41%
Yilmaz [20]	34	2004	85%	72%
Alsoufi [3]	174	2006	75%	61%
Akay [9]	157	2006	83%	73%
Han [10]	871	2007	75%	63%
Pagni [53]	131	2013	75%	45%

X- CONCLUSION

Triple mitro-aortic and tricuspid valve disease still occupies an important place in cardiac pathology in our country. This is due to the persistence of AAR, which poses a major public health problem. Surgical treatment is the gold standard. However, indications, surgical techniques and long-term results remain controversial.A review of the literature has shown that the mortality rate for trivalvular surgery is between 9% and 17% (pathology with a poor prognosis).Early mortality factors have been identified in most published articles [9, 10]. Nevertheless, LV DTD > 50 mm and age > 50 years were retained as early mortality factors by Akay [9] and Carrier [4] respectively. The actuarial survival published by Akay [9] and Yilmaz [20] was 82% and 74% at 5 and 10 years respectively. However, these survival rates found by Carrier [4], Alsoufi [3], Han [10] and Pagni [53] were lower. The factors that influence long-term survival are redux surgery and LV dysfunction (LVEF < 50%). The De Vega technique is often preferred by certain teams [3, 9, 10, 43] due to the speed with which it can be performed. This saves time, particularly during aortic clamping. Other teams [44] prefer prosthetic annuloplasty because of its greater durability. Finally, the rheumatic aetiology of triple valve disease is still predominant in developing countries, which presents a major public health problem. This has prompted a reassessment of the national programme to combat AAR in order to reduce the incidence of this serious disease. In addition, a better understanding of the risk factors for morbidity and mortality and proper patient selection will help to reduce the mortality rate.

BIBLIOGRAPHY

1. Tankut HA, Bahadir G, Süleyman O, et al. Triple-valve procedures: impact of risk on midterm in a rheumatic population. Ann Thorac Surg, 2006; 82: 1729-34.

2. Ministry of Public Health. Programme National de prévention et de lutte contre le rhumatisme cardiaque. Situation épidémiologique, 2008; p.2.

3. Alsoufi B, Rao V, Borger MA, et al. Short- and long-term results of triple valve surgery in the modern era. Ann Thorac Surg, 2006; 81: 2172-8.

4. Carrier M, Pellerin M, Bouchard D, et al. Long-term results with triple valve surgery. Ann Thorac Surg, 2002; 73: 44-7.

5. Filsoufi F, Fuzellier J.F, Fabiani J.N. Chirurgie des lésions acquises de la valve mitrale (I). EMC Techniques chirurgicales-Thorax, 1998; 42-531: 34p.

6. Leguerrier A, Langanay T, Vola M. Surgery for acquired aortic valve lesions. EMC Techniques chirurgicales-Thorax, 2007; 42-570: 35p.

7. Chauvaud S. Surgery for acquired tricuspid valve lesions. EMC Techniques chirurgicales-Thorax, 2002; 42-540: 8p.

8. Mullany CJ, Gersh BJ et al. Repair of tricuspid valve insufficiency in patients undergoing double (aortic and mitral) valve resplacement. J Thorac Cardiovasc Surg, 1987; 94: 740-8.

9. Akay TH, Gultekin B, Ozkan S et al. Triple calves procedures: Impact of risk factors on midterm in a rheumatic population. Ann Thorac Surg, 2006; 82: 1729.

10. Han QQ. Xu ZY, Zou LJ et al. Primary triple valve surgery for advanced rheumatic heart disease in Mainland China: a single-center experience with 871 clinical cases. Eur J cardiothorac Surg, 2007; 31: 845-50.

11. Eukouhen D. Advanced valvular heart disease: Prise en charge chirurgicale (à propos de 59 cas) service de chirurgie cardio-vasculaire du centre hospitalier universitaire Ibn Rochd, 2007; 48.

12. Michel P.L, Elias. Retrecissement. In Acar J, Acar C. Acquired valvular heart disease. Medecine-Sciences, Flammarion, 2000; 242-8.

13. Michel P.L, Abou Jaoud S. Triscupid insufficiency. In Acar J, Acar C, Cardiopathies valvulaires acquises. Medecine-Sciences, Flammarion, 2000; 249-61.

14. Porte J.-M Porte, Checrallah and Acar J. Mitral narrowing. In Acar J, Acar, Cardiopathies valvulaires acquises. Medecine-Sciences, Flammarion, 2000; 147-69.

15. Luxereau P, Michel P.L. Aortic insufficiency. In Acar J, Acar C, Cardiopathies valvulaires acquises. Medecine-Sciences, Flammarion, 2000; 222-41.

16. Gash AK, Carabello BA, Kent RL, Frazier JA, Spann JF. Left ventricular performance in patients with coexistent mitral stenosis and aotic insufficiency. J Am Coll Cardiol 1984; 3: 703-11.

17. Bonow et al. 2008 focused update incorporated into the ACC/AHA 2006 Guidelines for the management of patients with valvular heart disease. Circulation 2008; 118: 523-661.

18. Kirklin JW, Barrat-Boyes BG. Cardiac Surgery, 2nd Ed. New York, Churchill-Livingstone, 1993.

19. Hanania G, Maroni J-P, Terdjman M. Polyvalvulopathies. In Acar J, Acar C, Cardiopathies valvulaires acquises. Médecine-Sciences, Flammarion, 2000; 263-73.

20. Di Matteo J, Vacheron A, Lefeuvre C. Cardiologie, 3rd edition, 1999, Expansion scientifique Publications.

21. De Paepe A, Devereux RB, Dietz HC et al. Revised diagnostic criteria for the Marfan syndrome. Am J Hum Genet, 1996; 62: 417-26.

22. Acar J, Luxereau P. Indications opératoires et valvulopthies acqyuises. Arch Mal coeur, 1981; 74: 249-53.

23. Goutandji Ange G.H. Romuald M. Surgical management of triple valve disease. 2013; 123.

24. Garg SK, Gosh PK, Misra B. Triple valve surgery in rheumatic heart disease cardiologie tropicale, 1998; 24(94): 39-45.

25. Aubert S., Rubin S., Ouattara A., Bors V., Bonnet N., Leprince P., Gandjbakhch I., Pavie
A. Iterative cardiac surgery: from sternotomy to cannulation. EMC (Elsevier Masson SAS, Paris), Techniques chirurgicales - Thorax, 2008; 42-516.

26. Campos J-M, Paniagua P. Hypothermia during cardiac surgery. Best practice & research clinical anaesthesiology, 2008; 22(4): 695-709.

27. Vazquez-Jimenez JF, Qing M, Hermanns M, et al. Moderate hypothermia during cardiopulmonary bypass reduces myocardial cell damage and myocardial cell death related to cardiac surgery. J Am Coll Card 2001; 38(4): 1216-23.

28. Obadia J.-F, Chassignol J.-F. Mitral valve replacement. In Acar J, Acar C. Acquired valvular heart disease. Medecine-Sciences, Flammarion, 2000; 406-15.

29. Fuzellier JF, Filsoufi F, Berrebi A and Fabiani JN. Surgery for acquired mitral valve lesions (II). Encycl Med Chir (Elsevier, Paris), Techniques chirurgicales-Thorax, 1999; 42-531: 14p.

30. Acar C, Tapia M. Mitral plastic surgery. In Acar J, Acar C. Acquired valvular heart disease. Medecine-Sciences, Flammarion, 2000; 393-405.

31. Michal Šmíd et al. Mild to Moderate Functional Tricuspid Regurgitation: Retrospective Comparison of Surgical and Conservative Treatment. Research Cardiology Research and Practice 2010; 5p.

32. Chauvaud S. Surgery for acquired tricuspid valve lesions. EMC (Elsevier Masson SAS, Paris), Techniques chirurgicales - Thorax, 2009; 42-540.

33. Grondin P, Meere C, Limet R, Lopez-Bescoc L, Delcan JL, Rivera R. Carpentier's annulus and De Vega's annuloplasty. The end of the tricuspid challenge. J Thorac Cardiovasc Surg, 1975; 70: 852-9.

34. Limayem F, Carrier M, Vanderperren O, Petitclerc R, Pelletier LC. Comparative, clinical and echocardiographic study of the Bex and De Vega annuloplasties. Arch Mal Coeur 1991; 84: 937-41.

35. Abe T, Tukamoto M, Yanagiya M et al. De Vega's annuloplasty for acquired tricuspid disease: Early and late results in 110 patients. Ann thorac Surg, 1996; 62: 876-7.

36. Holper K, Haehnel JC, Augustin N et al. Surgery for tricuspid insufficiency: long-term follow-up after De Vega annuloplasty. Thorac Cardiovasc Surg, 1993; 41: 1-8.

37. Shahani R, Magotra RA. Late Follow-up of tricuspid valve replacement for unguarded tricuspid annulus. J Thorac Cardiovasc Surg, 1996; 112: 555-6.

38. Chauvaud S. Tricuspid valve surgery. In Acar J, Acar C. Acquired valvular heart disease. Medecine-Sciences, Flammarion, 2000; 433-7.

39. Guerra F, Bortolotti U, Thiene G, et al. Long-term performance of the Hancock porcine bioprosthesis in the tricuspid position. A review of forty-five patients with fourteen-year follow- up. J Thorac Cardiovasc Surg, 1990; 99: 838-45.

40. Coll MJ, Jegaden O, Janoby P, Rumolo A, Bonnefoy JY, Mikaeloff P. Results of triple valve replacement: perioperative mortality and long-term results. J Cardiovasc Surg 1987; 28: 369- 73.

41. Nakano K, Koyanagi H, Hashimoto A, Ohtsuka G, Nojiri C. Tricuspid valve replacement with the bileaflet St. Jude Medical valve prosthesis. J Thorac Cardiovasc Surg, 1994; 108: 888-92.

42. Horstkotte D, Schulte HD, Bircks W, Strauer BE. Lower intensity anticoagulation therapy results in lower complication rates with the St. Jude Medical prosthesis. J Thorac Cardiovasc Surg, 1994; 107: 1136-45.

43. Shinn HO S, Young Na et al Short- and Long-Term Results of Triple Valve Surgery: A Single Center Experience J Korean Med Sci, 2009; 24: 818-23.

44. Alec Vahanian et al. Guidelines on the management of valvular heart disease (2012 version). European Heart Journal, 2012; 33: 2451-96.

45. 2014/ACC Guideline for the Management of Patients With Valvular Heart Disease Journal of the American College of Cardiology 2014 by the American Heart Association, Inc. and the American College of Cardiology Foundation Published by Elsevier Inc.

46. Gersh BJ, Schaff HV, Vatterott PJ, et al. Results of triple valve replacement in 91 patients: perioperative mortality and long-term follow-up. Circulation, 1985; 72: 130-7.

47. Macmanus Q, Grunkemeier G, Starr A. Late results of triple valve replacement: a 14-year review. Ann Thorac Surg, 1978; 25: 402-6.

48. Bourezak SE, Chauvaud S, Romano M, Carpentier A. Triple valve replacement. Assessment of 90 patients operated. Arch Mal Cœur, 1984; 7: 724-9.

49. Donald GM, Kattus A, Davis CD, Drinkwater W. Long-term survival after triple valve replacement. Ann Thorac Surg, 1989; 48: 289-91.

50. Bortolotti U, Milano A, Testolin L. Influence of type of prosthesis on late results after combined mitro-aortic valve replacement. Ann Thorac Surg, 1991; 52: 84-91.

51. Brown PS, Roberts CS, Macintosh J, et al. Late results after triple valve replacement with various substitute valves. Ann Thorac Surg, 1993; 55: 5028.

52. John S, Ravikumar E, Colin JN, et al. 25-year experience with 456 combined mitral and aortic valve replacement for rheumatic heart disease. Ann Thorac Surg, 2000; 69: 1167-72.

53. Pagni S, Ganzel BL, Singh R, et al. Clinical outcome after triple-valve operations in the modern era: are elderly patients at increased surgical risk? Ann Thorac Surg 2013; Article in press.

54. Stephenson LW, Kouchoukos NT, Kirklin JW. Triple-valve replacement: an analysis of eight years' experience. Ann Thorac Surg, 1977; 23: 327-32.

55. Fadel BM, Alsoufi B, Manlhiot C, et al. Determinants of short- and long-term outcomes following triple valve surgery. J Heart Valve Dis, 2010; 19: 513-22.

TABLE OF CONTENTS

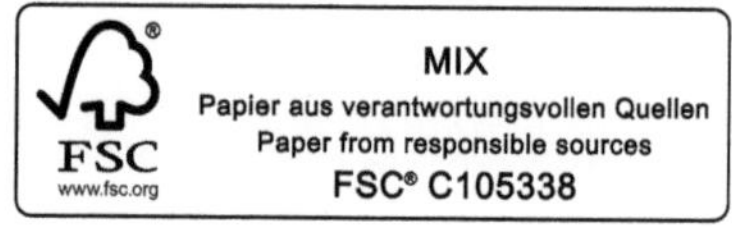

Printed by Books on Demand GmbH, Norderstedt / Germany